HEART VISION

:: JOURNAL ::

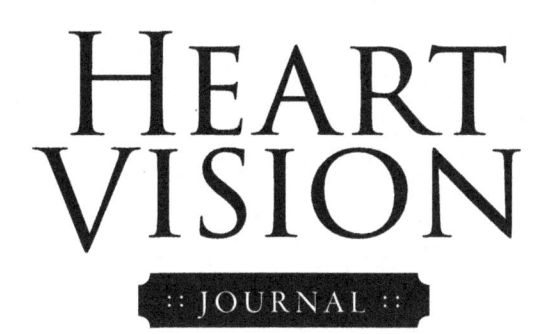

This ***Heart Vision Journal*** belongs to:

_____

"Look with your eyes under the brightest light, through the perfect lens for the infinite view."
—**Dr. Dellia Evans**

BONUS MATERIAL INSIDE

This journal contains prayers, scriptures, heart reflections, and extra activities to put your faith into action that are not included in the *Heart Vision* book

HEART VISION

:: JOURNAL ::

How to See Your Path Forward
When You're in a Dark Place

Dr. Dellia Evans

Copyright © 2019 by Dr. Dellia Evans

All rights reserved. This book or any portion thereof may not be reproduced or used in any manner whatsoever without the express written permission of the publisher except for the use of brief quotations in a book review.

ISBN 978-1-7341287-3-4

Cover and Interior Design by Jerry Dorris
Edited by Madalyn Stone

First Printing 2019
Butterflies Publishing
Jackson, MS 39236

For more information on buying this book in bulk, please email visible@drdellia.com.

Printed in the United States of America

A NOTE FROM THE AUTHOR

If you feel you are in a threatening environment, and you feel uncomfortable doing any of the challenges in the **Shine Your Light** exercises, please use your discretion.

—Dr. Dellia Evans

HEART VISION JOURNAL

There are seven chapters in *Heart Vision*. In the first six chapters, I reveal blind spots that can keep you stuck in a destructive marriage or intimate partner abusive relationship. Your relationship with your partner may be quite distant or over at this point. Regardless of where you find yourself, journaling can help you with self-awareness, action steps, and the healing process. The last chapter is about moving forward toward your purpose.

Use your *Heart Vision Journal* to see the reality of your situation even better. Then you will be empowered to make the best decision for yourself and your children. If you would like to read one chapter in *Heart Vision* per week, consider using *Heart Vision* along with your *Heart Vision Journal* to help you reflect God in your life daily. *Heart Vision* and your *Heart Vision Journal* can also help you to grow spiritually over the next two months.[*]

You can use your *Heart Vision Journal* to write down your thoughts, and what God will lay on your heart as you read and reflect. This will help you to remember these things better and stay accountable to yourself. Journaling can help you to have better spiritual vision. It helps you to be more focused as you look with your heart to see what you need to do concerning your marriage or intimate relationship.

I encourage you to make a commitment to read each chapter over a two-day period and to journal the next five days each week. You can use your *Heart Vision Journal* time as your daily devotional quiet time with God to get to know

---

[*] If you want to make sure your heart is in fellowship with God, before you start this spiritual journey, you can find a simple prayer in appendix C of *Heart Vision* to help you with this. After committing your heart to God with this prayer, you will be able to see with your heart more clearly what He would have you to do concerning your relationship with your partner and moving forward towards a brighter future.

yourself and Him better. As you think about your marriage and follow this MAP, I will direct you in prayer, guide you to read certain Bible verses (or scriptures), encourage you to SEE inside your heart, and challenge you to take action steps of faith for yourself and your marriage.

There are 3-4 additional pages for writing notes at the end of each week for extra journaling. Use these pages to write whatever you want. You may use it if you need more space to answer a question or if you have an idea or personal thoughts that you want to remember. In this note section, write your plans and/or impressions that God gives you in your spirit that week.

For an even closer relationship with God, I challenge you to make a commitment to memorize one scripture a week. Decide which one of five scriptures you will memorize each week. Write that scripture on a piece of paper, and put it in a place where you will continue to see it during the week (your bathroom mirror, your nightstand, the screen saver on your computer, the wallpaper of your cell phone, or the dashboard of your car, etc.)

Say this scripture to yourself out loud so you can hear it over and over. When you do this exercise, you are doing what Joshua 1:8 speaks about. If I paraphrase this scripture, it means to meditate on the Word of God day and night so that you will have good success. By memorizing scripture like this, you will also be doing what Psalm 119:11 says when it talks about hiding the Word of God in your heart.

So, let's get started journaling!

PART 1

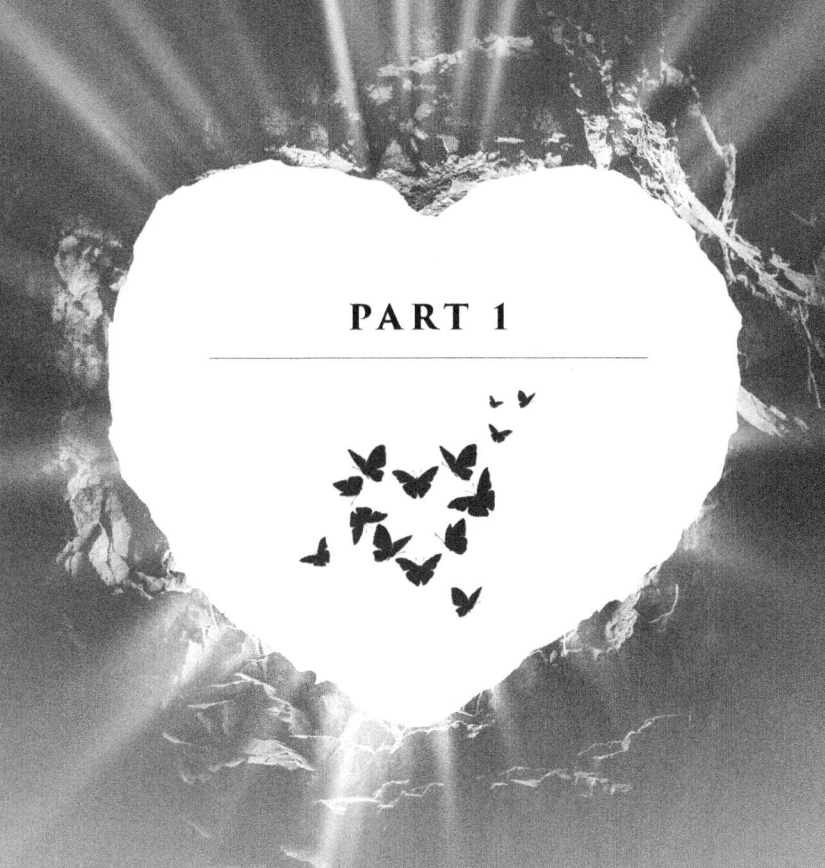

M.A.P.
Your Divine Reflection

WEEK 1

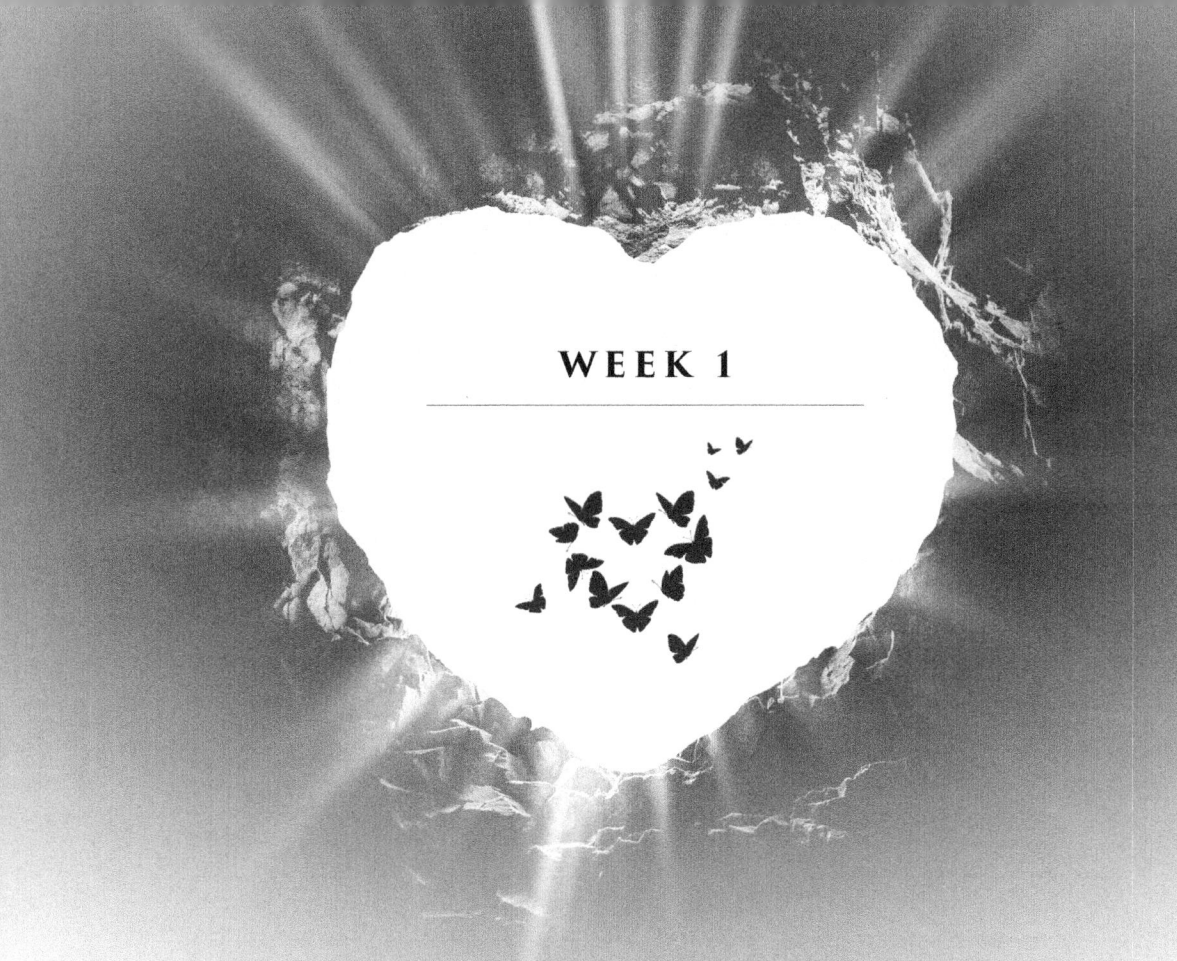

CHAPTER 1: M–Misinformation

HERE IS MY PRAYER FOR YOU THIS WEEK:

Father God, You are all-knowing and full of wisdom. Thank You for giving my sister Your wisdom and understanding for what You would have her to do in her life concerning her marriage. Give her Your viewpoint on how her choices are affecting her now and, in the future, and how they are affecting other people in her life. Help her to realize what a healthy relationship looks like. Lead her to a place where she can enjoy giving and receiving the fruit of the Spirit every day. Let her only agree with those who are in line with Your will. Help her to choose what brings life to her on every level of her well-being—spiritually, physically, emotionally, and financially. In Jesus' name I pray. Amen.

This week you will discover the best lens (or scriptures) to look through in the Bible so that you will not have spiritual myopic vision because of misinformation.

In prayer I will lead you to ask God to give you His eternal view, so that you will not be limited by the nearsightedness of limited understanding of His Word.

Hopefully, you will no longer have the blind spot of misinformation after reading this chapter that some women might have.

I will challenge you to do several things this week to let your light shine and to put your heart vision into motion.

In your journal look ahead at the **Perfect Lens** of **The Word** for the next five days. In the space provided, write the Bible verse that you chose for your scripture memory for this week:

_____
_____
_____
_____
_____
_____

Each day read your memory verse for the week first. Then read the scripture for that day before you pray.

DAY 1

GOD'S VIEWPOINT
The Big Picture

In the space below, write a personal prayer to Father God expressing your commitment to memorizing scriptures so that you will have His perspective.

Dear Father God,

_____
_____
_____
_____
_____
_____
_____
_____
_____

In Jesus' name

Amen

THE PERFECT LENS–THE WORD

Read James 1:5

If any of you lacks wisdom, you should ask God, who gives generously to all without fault, and it will be given to you.

HEART VISION

Close your eyes and look with your heart at what your personal home life looks like now. When you open your eyes, write what you saw in the space provided.

_____
_____
_____
_____

Are you being treated like God wants His daughter to be treated?

_____

If not, are you exhausted and tired of being treated like you are?

_____

Describe how you are being treated.

_____
_____
_____
_____
_____

How does that makes you feel?

_____

_____

_____

_____

Ask God to give you His wisdom as you make a decision to do what is best for you and possibly your children. If you are being led to do something different from what you are doing now, write it here. If not, write down that you will continue to keep your heart open to the leading of the Lord.

_____

_____

_____

_____

SHINE YOUR LIGHT

Who can you trust to talk to in order to get godly counsel if you are not being treated like God's daughter should be?

_____

Call and set up an appointment to talk to that person this week. Write the date and time of the appointment here:

_____

If you cannot think of anyone, look up a trusted resource in appendix B.

DAY 2

GOD'S VIEWPOINT
The Big Picture

In the space below, write a personal prayer to Father God asking Him to give you a clear understanding of His Word. This will help you not to be misinformed, and this will also help you to more effectively apply His Word to your life.

Father God,

_____

_____

_____

_____

_____

_____

_____

_____

In Jesus' name,

Amen

THE PERFECT LENS – THE WORD

Read Proverbs 4:7 ISV

Wisdom is of utmost importance, therefore get wisdom, and with all your effort work to acquire understanding.

HEART VISION

Close your eyes and look with your heart at what you want your personal home life to look like in three months. When you open your eyes, write what you saw in the space provided.

_____
_____
_____
_____

Are you agreeing to requests in your marriage that are not as the Lord would desire? If yes, how?

_____
_____
_____
_____

Why are you agreeing to these requests?

_____
_____
_____
_____

Ask God what He wants you to do concerning these requests. While you are still and quite before God in your quite time, what is He leading you to do? Write it down right here.

_____
_____
_____
_____
_____

SHINE YOUR LIGHT

If you are not being treated with respect in your marriage, what choice will you make to cause a positive change in your life?

_____
_____
_____
_____

What actions can you take to make this choice become a reality?

_____
_____
_____
_____

DAY 3

GOD'S VIEWPOINT
The Big Picture

In the space below, write your own personal prayer to Father God thanking Him for giving you the authority to use your own free will to make choices that will bring you and possibly your children new life.

Father God,

_____

_____

_____

_____

_____

_____

_____

In Jesus' name,

Amen

THE PERFECT LENS – THE WORD

Read Deuteronomy 30: 19 NIV

This day I call the heavens and the earth as witnesses against you that I have set before you, life and death, blessings and curses. Now choose life, so that you and your children may live.

HEART VISION

Close your eyes and look with your heart at what you want your personal home life to look like in six months. When you open your eyes, write what you saw in the space provided.

_____

_____

_____

_____

_____

Is your marriage honoring Christ and giving God glory?

_____

If not, what is the fruit that your marriage is producing if it is not the fruit of the Spirit?

_____

_____

_____

_____

Day 3

The fruit of the Spirit is love, peace, joy, kindness, gentleness, goodness, faithfulness, and moderation. Are there any of these fruit that your marriage is not producing that you want to be able to enjoy yourself?

_____

If so, list them below:

_____
_____
_____
_____

Ask God to show you what choices you have that will result in your life truly bringing glory to Him. In your quiet time, what is He showing you in your heart? Write it down right here.

_____
_____
_____
_____

SHINE YOUR LIGHT

What can you do to truly honor Christ when it comes to your marriage?

_____
_____
_____
_____

DAY 4

GOD'S VIEWPOINT
The Big Picture

In the space below, write your own personal prayer to Father God that you, *as His daughter, as the apple of His eye,* have some special requests of your Spiritual Daddy concerning your personal home life.

Father God,

_____

_____

_____

_____

_____

_____

_____

In Jesus' name,

Amen

THE PERFECT LENS – THE WORD

Read Psalm 37: 4 ISV

Delight yourself in the Lord, and He will give you the desires of your heart.

HEART VISION

Close your eyes and look with your heart at what *you* want *your* personal home life to look like in one year. When you open your eyes, write what you saw in the space provided.

_____
_____
_____

In your heart, what do you want for your marriage, your children, and your home?

_____
_____
_____

Make a list of the things that *you* want for *yourself*:

_____
_____
_____

Find a picture that symbolizes one thing that *you* want for *yourself*. Print or cut it out and put it somewhere that you can look at every day.

Thank God for giving you your heart's desire by faith before you receive it.

DAY 5

GOD'S VIEWPOINT
The Big Picture

In the space below, write your own personal prayer to Father God to let *His will* be done in your life in order to bring about the peace and love that He wants you to have.

Father God,

_____
_____
_____
_____
_____
_____
_____
_____

In Jesus' name,

Amen

THE PERFECT LENS – THE WORD

Read Luke 22: 42b NLT

Father... I want Your will to be done, not mine.

HEART VISION

Close your eyes and look with your heart at what *you* want *your* personal home life to look like in five years. When you open your eyes, write what you saw in the space provided.

_____
_____
_____
_____

If God's will for your life is different from yours, are you open to accepting that?

_____

If you are open, how can accepting God's will be better for you?

_____
_____
_____
_____

If not, why are you not open to accepting God's will?

_____

SHINE YOUR LIGHT

Write down the obstacles that are keeping you from experiencing the peace, love, happiness, respect, and freedom you and your children deserve.

_____
_____
_____
_____
_____

Is your life and the lives of your children worth what you would have to go through to overcome these obstacles?

_____

If you believe God cares about you enough, and loves you enough to see you through these obstacles, and that He is able and willing to provide your every need, what can you do to put your faith into motion?

_____
_____
_____
_____

Week 1 Notes

Week 1 Notes

WEEK 2

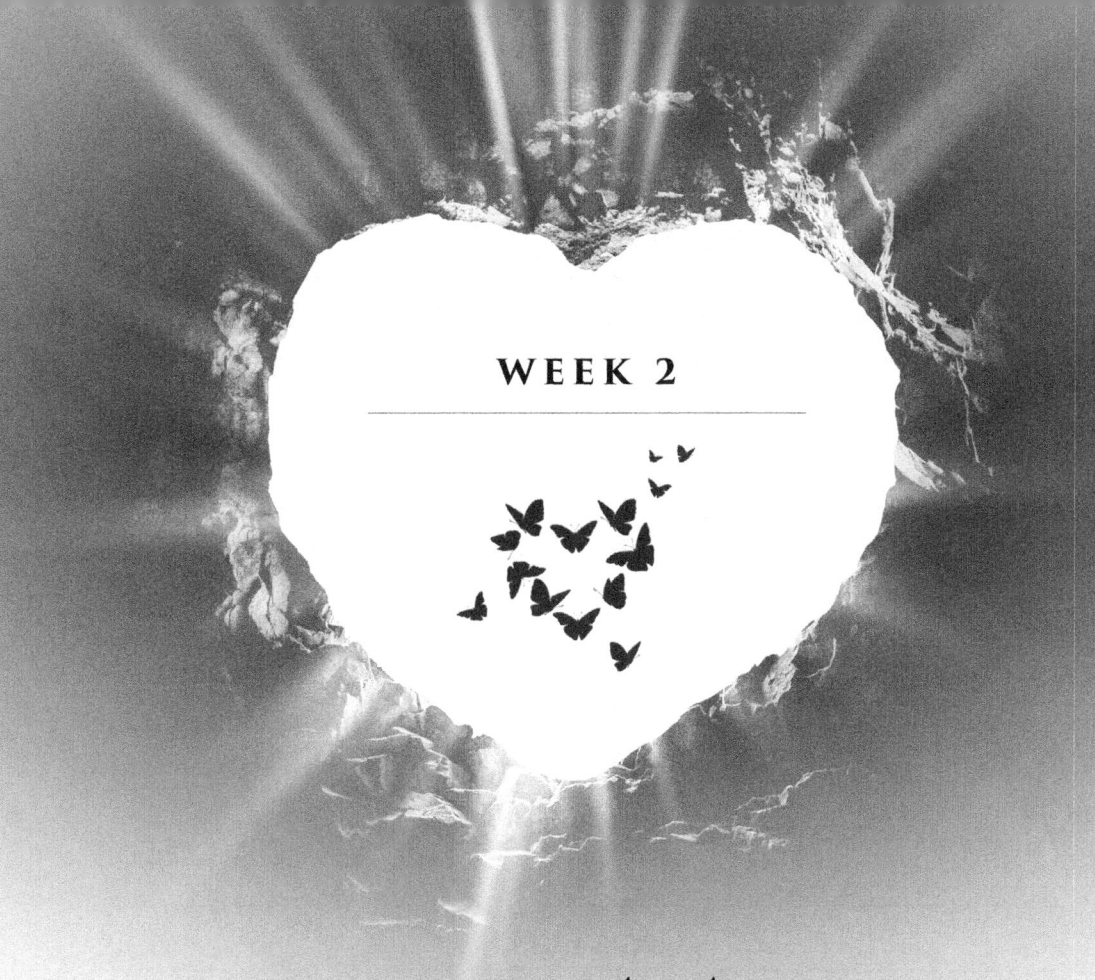

CHAPTER 2: A- Anxiety

HERE IS MY PRAYER FOR YOU THIS WEEK:

Father God, You are all powerful and our ever-present help in the time of trouble. I lift up my sister before You today. Thank you, God, for being her provider. Thank You, Jesus, for being her Prince of Peace, and thank You, Holy Spirit, for being her Comforter. I agree with Your Word that You have not given her the spirit of fear, but of power, love, and a strong mind. I thank You for giving her Your peace that will surpass her understanding and will keep her thoughts and her heart quiet, so that she will have peaceful rest.

I agree with my sister right now that: she trusts, depends, and has her confidence in You; she chooses to think on good thoughts; and she will not choose thoughts that will cause her to worry, fret, or allow her heart to be troubled.

Instead of worrying, she will pray to You about her concerns. And because her hope and expectancy are in You, Oh Lord, we thank You for the answers to her prayers in the way that You see fit. We thank You for providing all of her needs, and that she will not be in want. For this we will continue to give You our thanks and praise. In Jesus' name we pray. Amen

This week you will discover the best lens (or scriptures) to look through in the Word of God so that you can be delivered from worry and anxiety.

In prayer I will lead you to ask God to give you His eternal view, so that anxiety will not be the blind spot that limits your mobility.

I will challenge you to do several things this week to let your light shine and to put your heart vision into motion.

In your journal, look ahead at the **Perfect Lens** of **The Word** for the next five days. In the space provided, write the Bible verse that you chose for your scripture memory for this week:

_____

_____

_____

_____

Each day read your memory verse for the week first. Then read the scripture for that day before you pray.

DAY 6

GOD'S VIEWPOINT
The Big Picture

In the space below, write your own personal prayer to Father God to let your home be a place where every member of your family can rest. Ask Him to let it be a peaceful and safe place for you every day.

Father God,

_____
_____
_____
_____
_____
_____
_____
_____

In Jesus' name,

Amen

THE PERFECT LENS – THE WORD

Read Isaiah 32:18 NIV

My people will live in peaceful dwelling places, in secure homes, in undisturbed places of rest.

HEART VISION

Close your eyes and look with your heart at what your home looks like to you now and what a quiet and peaceful, safe home looks like to you in the future. When you open your eyes, write what you saw in the space provided.

_____
_____
_____
_____

Do you see any threats to you, or are your children in physical danger?

_____

If so, what are they?

_____
_____
_____
_____

Are you being hurt emotionally?

_____

If so, in what way?

___

What about being verbally, financially, or psychologically abused?

___

If so, in what way?

___

SHINE YOUR LIGHT

What can you do to have a beautiful, quiet, safe, peaceful home?

___

What area of your home can you start on to organize, clean, and/or clear clutter?

_____
_____
_____
_____

DAY 7

GOD'S VIEWPOINT
The Big Picture

In the space below, write your own personal prayer to Father God to reveal to you the heart of your husband towards you.

Father God,

_____

_____

_____

_____

_____

_____

_____

_____

In Jesus' name,

Amen

THE PERFECT LENS – THE WORD

Read Luke 6:45 NRS

The good person out of the good treasure of the heart produces good, and the evil person out of evil treasure produces evil; for it is out of the abundance of the heart that the mouth speaks.

HEART VISION

Close your eyes and look with your heart at how your husband's hurtful actions and words have affected you and your children. When you open your eyes, write what you saw and felt.

_____
_____
_____
_____
_____
_____

How does your husband consistently show that he wants to make changes to create a healthy relationship with you, addressing your needs and concerns?

_____
_____
_____
_____
_____
_____

Is he willing to get help from a counselor trained in diagnosing and treating abusers in domestic violence cases?

_____
_____

Are you willing to go to counseling (with or without your husband) to learn what you can do to take care of yourself so that you can find healing?

_____

Shine Your Life

If you and your husband are willing, make an appointment with a behavioral health therapist trained in domestic violence cases. Find a counselor through the resources in Appendix B. Write the appointment details here.

_____
_____

If the breach of the relationship is beyond counseling or counseling is not an option, what will you do to move on?

_____
_____
_____
_____
_____
_____

DAY 8

GOD'S VIEWPOINT
The Big Picture

In the space below, write your own personal prayer to Father God to free you from the fear of disapproval, so that other's opinions don't keep you from moving forward to your best life.

Father God,

_____

_____

_____

_____

_____

_____

_____

_____

In Jesus' name,

Amen

THE PERFECT LENS – THE WORD

Read Isaiah 61:1b NIV

He has sent Me to bind up the brokenhearted, to proclaim freedom for the captives and release from darkness for the prisoners.

HEART VISION

Close your eyes and look with your heart to see if you have closed it off to others outside of your marriage that could be a support to you to help you. When you open your eyes, write the names of the people that you saw.

_____

_____

_____

_____

What concerns do you have about other peoples' opinions of you?

_____

_____

_____

What do you feel is God's opinion of you?

_____

_____

_____

SHINE YOUR LIGHT

What can you do to be true to yourself and not give others who are close to you a false impression?

_____

_____

_____

_____

_____

_____

DAY 9

GOD'S VIEWPOINT
The Big Picture

In the space below, write your own personal prayer to Father God thanking Him for His faithfulness and provision so that you will not worry.

Father God,

_____

_____

_____

_____

_____

_____

_____

_____

In Jesus' name,

Amen

THE PERFECT LENS – THE WORD

Read Matthew 7:7-8 NIV

Ask, and it will be given to you; seek, and you will find; knock and it will be opened to you. For everyone who asks receives, and the one who seeks finds, and to the one who knocks it will be opened.

HEART VISION

Close your eyes and look with your heart to see how you want to be loved by your husband. When you open your eyes, write down what you saw.

_____
_____
_____
_____

In what ways do you feel loved by your husband?

_____
_____
_____
_____

What are the ways that you would like to be loved and have a sense of security that is missing now?

_____
_____
_____

SHINE YOUR LIGHT

If you are not being loved like you deserve to be, if you are just waiting on God, and not actively asking, knocking, and seeking what action He wants you to take, will you go online and order a ROUND TUIT today?

_____
_____

(Your ROUND TUIT will remind you to stop making excuses.)

God is waiting on you to use your free will to make a choice to step out on faith and trust Him to take care of you and your children. Do you believe this?

_____
_____

Well, what are you going to do about it? and when?

_____
_____
_____
_____
_____

DAY 10

GOD'S VIEWPOINT
The Big Picture

In the space below, write your own personal prayer to Father God to give you peace of mind about everything that *you* have to do that causes you to be stressed out.

Father God,

_____

_____

_____

_____

_____

_____

_____

_____

In Jesus' name,

Amen

THE PERFECT LENS – THE WORD

Read Philippians 4:6,19 NLT

Don't worry (or be anxious) about anything; instead pray about everything. Tell God what you need and thank Him for (what) He has done...And this same God who takes care of me will supply all your needs from His glorious riches, which have been given to us in Christ Jesus.

HEART VISION

Close your eyes and look with your heart to see what you can do and who you can ask for help and simplify your day. When you open your eyes, write down what you saw?

_____
_____
_____

Do you feel as if you are trying to fix your marriage alone?

_____

What all are you doing?

_____
_____

How would you like your husband to help?

_____
_____
_____

Based on how things currently are, do you really see that happening?

_____

SHINE YOUR LIGHT

Whom can you reach out to who will help you with your personal finances?

_____
_____

Will you look up government agencies, associations, and "Financial Peace" classes near you?

_____

What did you find out?

_____
_____
_____

Week 2 Notes

Week 2 Notes

WEEK 3

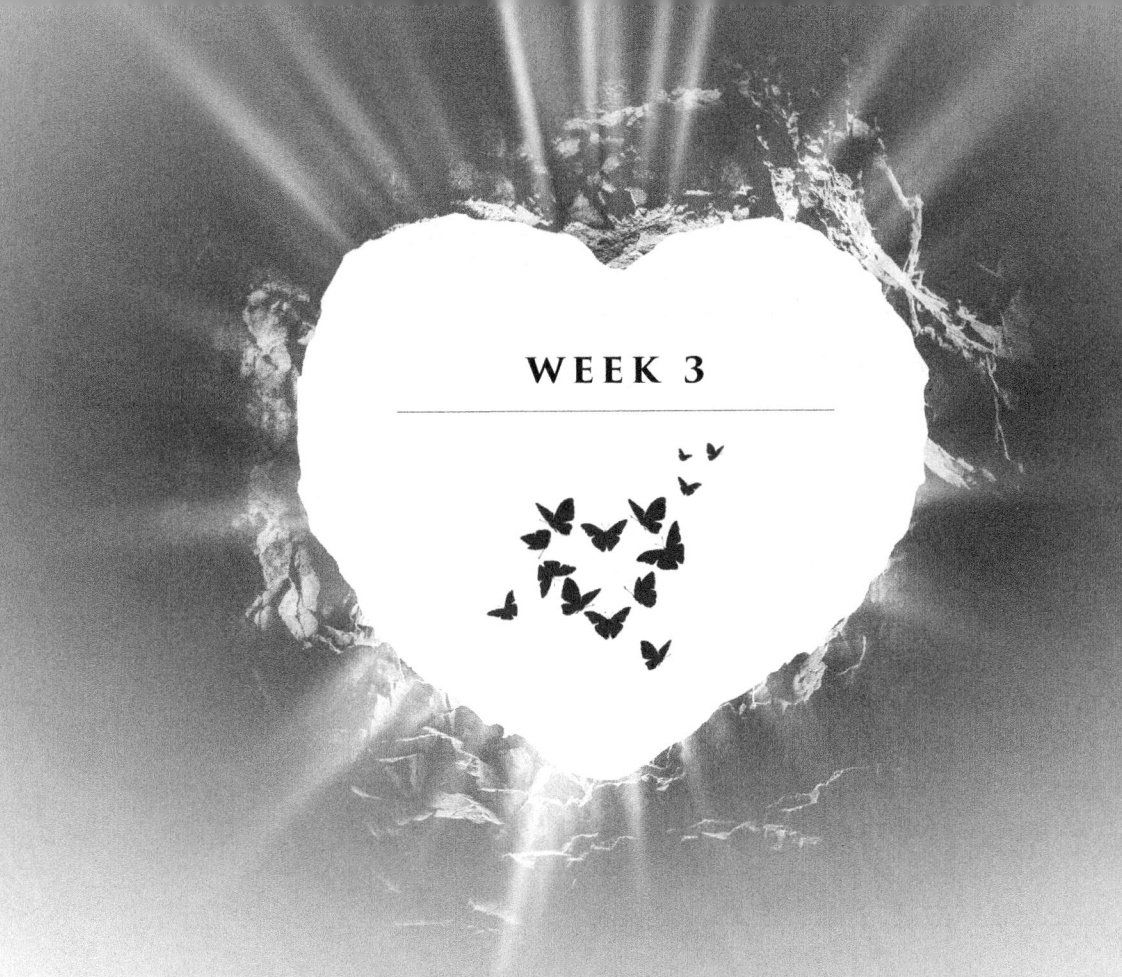

CHAPTER 3: P- Perception

HERE IS MY PRAYER FOR YOU THIS WEEK:

Father God, You alone are holy, and You know everything about my sister. You desire that she is truthful and honest in the inward parts of her heart. Help her to be honest with herself so that she can identify what is going on in her life and what she wants for herself and her family.

Help her to make wise decisions for her life. Help her to know how precious she is in your sight, how much You love her with Your everlasting love, and that You will see that her needs are met. Let her be open to the people that You will send across her path that will give her Your wise counsel, lift her up, and help her. All these things I ask in Jesus' name. Amen

This week you will discover the best lens (or scriptures) to look through in the Word of God so that you will not be limited by the tunnel vision that can come from your perception and the perception of others.

I will lead you in prayer to God so that you will receive the perception that He has of you. Ask Him for His eternal view so that you will not have any problem seeing the people in your peripheral vision.

Hopefully, by the time you finish reading this chapter, you will learn how your perception or other people's perceptions could be a blind spot that could limit your ability to move forward. By identifying this potential obstacle, you can then consider what you can do about it.

I will challenge you to do several things this week to let your light shine and put your heart vision into motion.

In your journal, look ahead at the **Perfect Lens** of **The Word** for the next five days. In the space provided, write the Bible verse that you chose for your scripture memory for this week:

_____

_____

_____

_____

_____

Each day read your memory verse for the week first. Then read the scripture for that day before you pray.

DAY 11

GOD'S VIEWPOINT
The Big Picture

In the space below, write your own personal prayer to Father God that He shows you how special you are to Him. Ask Him to help you see yourself through His eyes.

Father God,

_____

_____

_____

_____

_____

_____

_____

In Jesus' name,

Amen

THE PERFECT LENS – THE WORD

Read what God said about you, as His child, in Exodus 19:5 ESV

"Now therefore, if you will indeed obey My voice and keep My covenant, you shall be My treasured possession among all peoples, for all the Earth is Mine;"

HEART VISION

Close your eyes and look with your heart to see how your perception of yourself and others' perceptions of you are contributing to where you are today on your life's journey. When you open your eyes, in the space provided write what you saw.

_____
_____
_____
_____
_____
_____

Describe yourself. Do you perceive yourself as valuable, or do you doubt your own value? Why or Why not?

_____
_____
_____
_____
_____

SHINE YOUR LIGHT

Do something special for yourself because you deserve it. What will it be?

_____

_____

_____

When this week will you do it?

_____

_____

DAY 12

GOD'S VIEWPOINT
The Big Picture

In the space below, write your own personal prayer to Father God that He daily cleans your heart and that even though you have been mistreated, He helps you to continue to do the things in your life that finds favor in His sight.

Father God,

_____
_____
_____
_____
_____
_____
_____

In Jesus' name,

Amen

THE PERFECT LENS – THE WORD

Read 2 Timothy 2:15a (NLT)

Work hard so you can present yourself to God and receive His approval.

HEART VISION

Take a deep breath. This exercise will not be easy, but you can do it if you really want things to change. Close your eyes and look with your heart to see the painful things that you decided to endure at your own expense for the sake of your marriage. What things are you embarrassed about and don't want people to know that are going on in your life or home? When you open your eyes, in the space provided write down what you saw.

_____
_____
_____
_____
_____
_____

What is the single most troubling thing that you don't like about how your husband treats you and/or your children?

_____
_____
_____
_____

How do you feel about how your husband treats you and your children?

_____

_____

_____

_____

_____

SHINE YOUR LIGHT

Think of another person besides the one you mentioned on Day 1, whom you can trust. Think of a person who won't judge you, and whom you feel you can pray with and talk to about your marriage. Write their name here:

_____

Make an appointment this week to talk to this person. Write the place and time of the appointment here:

_____

When you make the appointment let them know that you want your conversation to be confidential (whatever you are comfortable sharing about what is going on with you in your marriage). Tell this individual that you are not looking for advice but just someone to listen and support you. Ask them to pray with you, that you make the best decision concerning your marriage.

If you cannot think of another person, look up a different trusted resource in appendix B.

DAY 13

GOD'S VIEWPOINT
The Big Picture

In the space below, write your own personal prayer to Father God that He allows you to be more sensitive to other women and men who may be in a toxic relationship.

Father God,

_____

_____

_____

_____

_____

_____

_____

_____

In Jesus' name,

Amen

THE PERFECT LENS – THE WORD

Read I Thessalonians 5:11 NLT

So, encourage each other and build each other up, just as you are already doing.

HEART VISION

Close your eyes and look in your heart and see yourself pretending to be okay concerning your marriage. How does it feel on the inside if you are pretending for days, weeks, months, and even years at a time? When you open your eyes, in the space provided write what you saw and felt.

_____

_____

_____

_____

Now, imagine if you were a guy being mistreated by your wife or girlfriend. He may feel like there is nothing that he can do. Sometimes men feel even more hopeless than women. Imagine trying to look tough on the outside, but on the inside his heart is the same as what you just wrote about in the above heart vision exercise. What could you say to this man to encourage him to get help or move on if his partner refuses to change?

_____

_____

_____

_____

SHINE YOUR LIGHT

Look for a man (among your family, friends, and coworkers) who may need you to encourage him to seek help if he is in a toxic relationship. When you come across this man who is usually suffering from emotional, psychological, verbal, and/or financial abuse from his partner, write his name here:

_____

Make a point to encourage him, pray for him, and offer him the resources for men in appendix B.

DAY 14

GOD'S VIEWPOINT
The Big Picture

In the space below, write your own personal prayer to Father God that you are able to perceive your own beauty both on the inside in your heart and on the outside.

Father God,

_____

_____

_____

_____

_____

_____

_____

In Jesus' name,

Amen

THE PERFECT LENS – THE WORD

Read Psalm 45:11a (GNT)

Your beauty will make the king desire you.

HEART VISION

Close your eyes and look in your heart and see your heart being quiet, peaceful, loving, cheerful, gentle, and kind. Imagine this beautiful heart giving off a radiant light that illuminates your whole body. Now imagine yourself getting all dolled up from head to toe. When you open your eyes, in the space provided write down what you saw and felt.

_____
_____
_____
_____
_____
_____
_____

When do you remember feeling like this?

_____
_____

Do you feel like you have to be in a relationship with someone to take pride in yourself and put forth extra effort in to look your best?

_____

Why or Why not?

_____
_____
_____

SHINE YOUR LIGHT

Within the next two days, have a date with yourself (even if you stay at home). Write down the time and place it will be here:

_____
_____
_____
_____

Be creative. Think of the things you like. (i.e. candles, flowers, strawberries, chocolates, popcorn, Netflix, etc.) Celebrate how wonderful and beautiful you are. Get dolled up. Take a selfie. Don't talk yourself out of it. Tell a friend or support person about your date.

Ask them to keep you accountable.

After your date, in the space available write down what you did, your thoughts, how you looked, how you felt (the good, the bad, the neutral).

_____
_____
_____
_____
_____

_____

_____

_____

*Share this **Shine Your Light** exercise and your selfie with your support person. Ask for their feedback.*

DAY 15

GOD'S VIEWPOINT
The Big Picture

In the space below, write your own personal prayer to Father God that you will be free from the fear of the approval of others.

Father God,

_____

_____

_____

_____

_____

_____

_____

_____

In Jesus' name,

Amen

THE PERFECT LENS – THE WORD

Read Galatians 1:10 (GNTD)

Does this sound as if I am trying to win human approval? No indeed! What I want is God's approval! Am I trying to be popular with people? If I were still trying to do so, I would not be a servant of Christ.

HEART VISION

Close your eyes and look in your heart and see yourself free from all forms of mistreatment. Then see the face of the very person that you did not want to ever find out about your abuse when you told them that you are now free. What is their response? When you open your eyes, in the space provided, write down the name of this person and what you saw and heard in your heart.

_____

_____

_____

_____

_____

Which is worse, staying silent and living a lifelong of disappointment and abuse and mistreatment, or sharing your story and facing this person's reaction and getting over it, and living free for the rest of your life?

_____

_____

_____

_____

Why did you answer this question the way that you did?

_____
_____
_____
_____
_____

How do you think others perceive you and your family now?

_____
_____
_____
_____
_____

Is this a true perception?

_____

Why or why not?

_____
_____
_____
_____
_____
_____

How do you feel about other people's perceptions of you and your family?

_____
_____
_____
_____
_____

What is more important to you, your temporary feelings or your permanent freedom?

_____
_____
_____
_____

SHINE YOUR LIGHT

Set aside fifteen minutes to look at Grace for Purpose's YouTube Video that was published on April 1, 2019. In this video, Lisa Bevere talks about perceptions—God's, yours, and others. It's called "You Are Worth More Than You Think, Woman of God." When can you look at it?

_____

Week 3 Notes

Week 3 Notes

PART 2

S.E.E.
Your Divine Reflection

WEEK 4

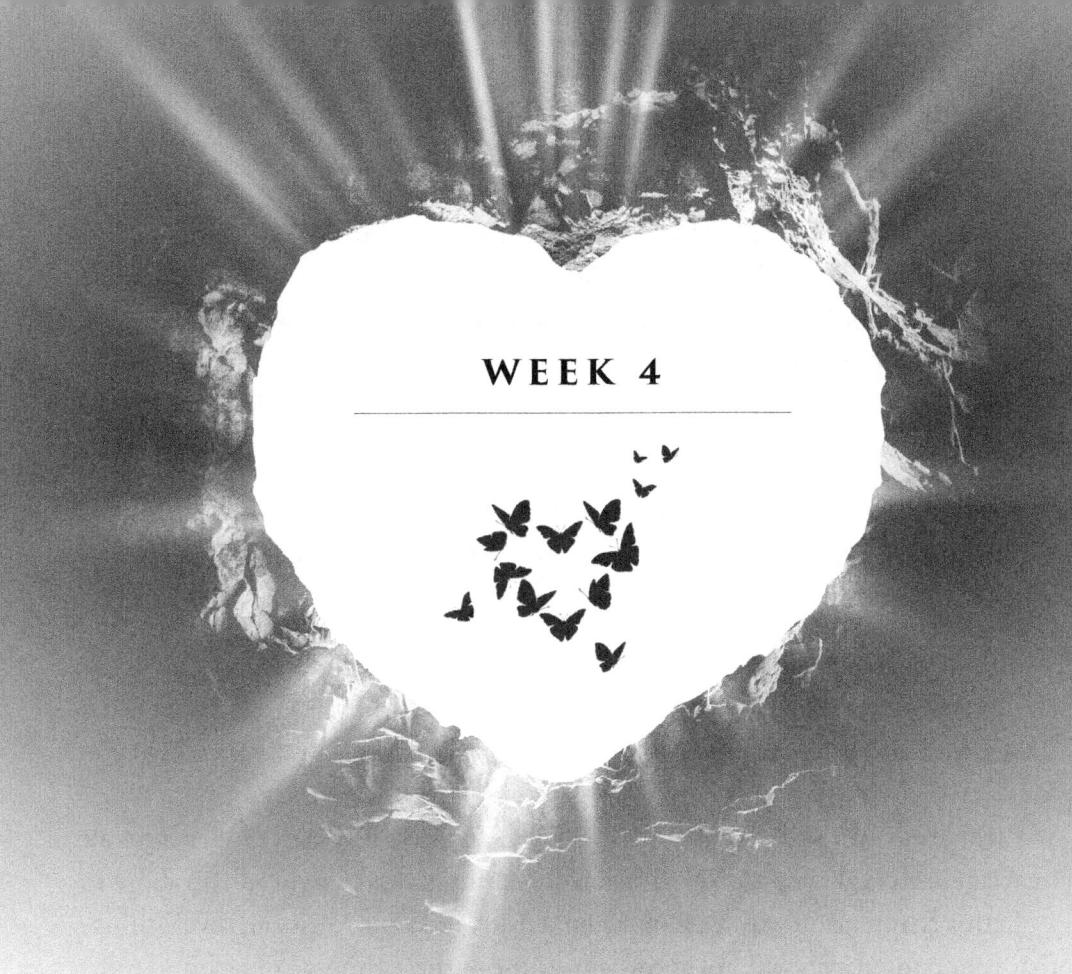

CHAPTER 4: S-Spirit

HERE IS MY PRAYER FOR YOU THIS WEEK:

Father God, You are sovereign. You are spirit. And we recognize who You are, and we honor You with our whole hearts. God, You see and search our hearts. Whatever You find that is not clean, we ask that You take it away and give us a clean heart. Renew a right spirit within us. From her clean heart, and her renewed spirit is the place where my sister connects with You, God.

Through faith, open the eyes of her heart so that she will see herself as You see her. Help her to see her life from Your perspective. Remind her of the wonderful dreams that You put in her heart years ago that You still want to manifest in her life. Show her the true fruit that her husband is or is not bearing from his spirit. Show her the spiritual fruit that You want her to enjoy.

Reveal any blind spots that she may have in her heart that she cannot see about herself. If she is being abused, let her see it for what it is. If she feels as if her life is in danger, protect her and help her to find a support person who will help her to establish a safe plan of escape. If she needs money to move forward with her plan to leave, show her what she needs to do so that You can help provide the financial assistance that is available to her.

Show her in Your Word and in her spirit the next steps that she should take daily concerning her marriage and family. All these things I ask in Jesus' name. Amen.

This week you will discover the best lens (or scriptures) to look through in the Word of God so that you will not only depend on your physical eyes to see what things really look like. Use this spiritual perspective to ground yourself as you look at the circumstances of your marriage with your spirit vision.

I will lead you to pray to God that He will give you His eternal view of your marriage and clarify your spiritual vision concerning what you should do about it.

In this chapter, you will see how being sensitive to your spirit can reveal things that your natural eyes will not show you. Some of these things can be blind spots that keep you from moving on in your life beyond abuse and into your purpose and can only be revealed by your spiritual vision.

I will challenge you to do several things this week to let your light shine and put your heart vision into motion.

In your journal, look ahead at the **Perfect Lens** of **The Word** for the next five days. In the space provided, write the Bible verse that you chose for your scripture memory for this week:

_____

_____

_____

_____

_____

Each day read your memory verse for the week first. Then read the scripture for that day before you pray.

DAY 16

GOD'S VIEWPOINT
The Big Picture

In the space below, write your own personal prayer to Father God that The Holy Spirit confirms in your heart that you are His daughter today. (If you are not sure, see the prayers in appendix C and follow my suggestions before doing this exercise.)

Father God,

_____
_____
_____
_____
_____
_____
_____
_____

In Jesus' name,

Amen

THE PERFECT LENS – THE WORD

Read Romans 8:16 NLT

For His Spirit joins with our spirit to affirm that we are God's children.

HEART VISION

Close your eyes and look at your new, cleansed heart that God has re-created. He has washed your heart clean by the blood of Jesus. When you open your eyes, in the space provided write what you saw.

_____

_____

_____

_____

_____

Are you now certain that your heart is connected to God so that you can communicate with each other freely?

_____

Why or why not?

_____

_____

_____

_____

_____

SHINE YOUR LIGHT

What can you do each day to make sure your spirit is in fellowship with God? (Again, see appendix C if you need help with this answer.)

___

Each day continue your devotional time after reading **Heart Vision**. There are many devotional books available at bookstores and online. Start looking for your next one today. Write down the name of the next devotional book that you will use after you finish **Heart Vision Journal.** Go ahead and purchase and/or order it now. Write down your purchase/order information here:

___

Read Lamentations 3:22-24 and thank God for new mercy every morning that He gives you to get you through the day.

DAY 17

GOD'S VIEWPOINT
The Big Picture

In the space below, write your own personal prayer to Father God that He helps you to use the eyes of your heart so that you can be led by your spiritual vision concerning your marriage.

Father God,

_____
_____
_____
_____
_____
_____
_____
_____

In Jesus' name,

Amen

THE PERFECT LENS – THE WORD

Read Ephesians 1:18 (Voice)

Open the eyes of their hearts and let the light of Your truth flood in. Shine Your light on the hope You are calling them to embrace. Reveal to them the glorious riches You are preparing as their inheritance.

HEART VISION

Close your eyes and look with your heart and see yourself free from the stress and mistreatment of an abusive partner. When you open your eyes in the space provided, write what you saw.

_____

_____

_____

SHINE YOUR LIGHT

Create what you saw in your heart vision exercise above. If you saw yourself at peace for example, **search** for scriptures that promise you peace. **Ask** God to give you these promises. **Write** these scriptures down. Use the power of your words! **Say** these scriptures out loud. Declare these promises as yours. **Thank** God for them before you get them as an act of your faith. Faith without works is dead. **Do what you can do** to make your spiritual vision in your heart vision exercise above a reality. **Expect** God to do the rest.

In the space provided write the scriptures that you will confess out loud: (i.e. Peace I leave with you; my peace I give you. I do not give to you as the world gives. Do not let you're your hearts be troubled and do not be afraid. John 14:27)

_____

_____

_____

DAY 18

GOD'S VIEWPOINT
The Big Picture

In the space below, write your own personal prayer to Father God that He will lead and guide you from your spirit through your faith. Ask God to help you to see things from His perspective as you make decisions concerning your marriage, children and plans to move forward. Ask Him to give you wisdom as you take action on your decisions.

Father God,

_____

_____

_____

_____

_____

_____

In Jesus' name,

Amen

The Perfect Lens – The Word

Read 2 Corinthians 5:7 (GW)

Indeed, our lives are guided by faith (eyes of faith, spiritual vision), not by sight (physical eyesight).

Heart Vision

Close your eyes and look in your heart so that you can see how healthy your spirit is on the inside. Does it look strong, cheerful, and growing, or does it look weak, sad, and crushed? When you open your eyes, write a detailed description of what you saw in the space provided.

_____
_____
_____
_____
_____

Why do you think your spirit looks like you just described?

_____
_____
_____

If you are a spirit, who has a soul (mind, emotion, and will), who lives in a body, you will make decisions and take action because one of these three parts of your being is the strongest at that moment. If your faith (spirit) is weak and you are more focused on your thoughts and emotions, your soul will guide your actions. If you are tired in your body and that is your focus, your body will lead your actions. If your faith is your strongest focus, your spirit can override your soul and your body.

Are you being led by your spirit, or are you allowing your soul (your thoughts and emotions) and how you feel in your body to lead you?

_____
_____

SHINE YOUR LIGHT

If your spirit is not leading you, which of the following will you make a commitment to do to build up your spirit? Mark which one you choose.

1) Choice One: Memorize and confess more scriptures concerning God's guidance and wisdom out loud so that you can hear yourself saying them.

_____

(i.e. Show me Your ways, Lord, teach me Your paths. Guide me in Your truth and teach me, for You are God my Savior, and my hope is in You all day long. Psalm 25:4-5) What other scriptures did you find?

_____
_____
_____

2) Choice Two: Talk more to God in prayer concerning what you should do and take more time to listen to what He says to you.

_____

When and How long?

_____

3) Choice Three: Stay in an atmosphere of praise with praise and worship music.

_____

What songs?

_____

DAY 19

GOD'S VIEWPOINT
The Big Picture

In the space below, write your own personal prayer to Father God that you will see a wonderful vision and dream for yourself in your bright future.

Father God,

_____

_____

_____

_____

_____

_____

_____

_____

_____

In Jesus' name,

Amen

The Perfect Lens – The Word

Read Proverbs 13:12b KJV

When dreams come true, there is life and joy.

Heart Vision

Close your eyes and look in your heart so that you can see the dream or vision that you want for your bright future. What good dream do you see for yourself and family with your partner? What good dream do you see for yourself and your family without your partner? When you open your eyes, write a detailed description of what you saw in the space provided.

_____
_____
_____
_____
_____

What dreams did you used to have in your heart for yourself that you have stopped dreaming about?

_____
_____
_____
_____

Will you start dreaming about them again?

_____

Why or why not?

_____
_____
_____

SHINE YOUR LIGHT

What can you do or to whom can you talk to help put you on the right track to making at least one of your dreams come true? If you want to talk to someone about this, who will it be? Write down who, when and where you will talk to them.

_____
_____
_____
_____
_____
_____

DAY 20

GOD'S VIEWPOINT
The Big Picture

In the space below, write your own personal prayer to Father God that you are not discouraged by what you see with your natural eyes in your relationship and your home right now. Ask God to help you to see the invisible, spiritual things that He has in store for you with your eyes of faith.

Father God,

_____

_____

_____

_____

_____

_____

_____

In Jesus' name,

Amen

THE PERFECT LENS – THE WORD

Read 2 Corinthians 4:18 (HCSB)

So, we do not focus on what is seen, but on what is unseen. For what is seen is temporary, but what is unseen is eternal.

HEART VISION

Close your eyes and look in your heart so that you can see why you are struggling with staying in your relationship even though you may be treated with disrespect. Look at why you want to stay. Look at why it may be best to leave. Are your children involved? What is best for you and your children in the long run? How can your relationship with your husband affect them when they become adults? When you open your eyes, write in detail what you saw in the space provided.

_____
_____
_____
_____
_____
_____

Do you feel like you are doing most of the work to make the relationship work?

_____

Why or Why not?

_____
_____
_____

What are the biggest challenges you have that would prevent you from deciding to get out of a relationship that is hurting you and your children?

_____
_____
_____
_____

Shine Your Light

What will you do to face one of the challenges that is causing you to stay where you are?

_____
_____
_____
_____
_____
_____

Week 4 Notes

Week 4 Notes

WEEK 5

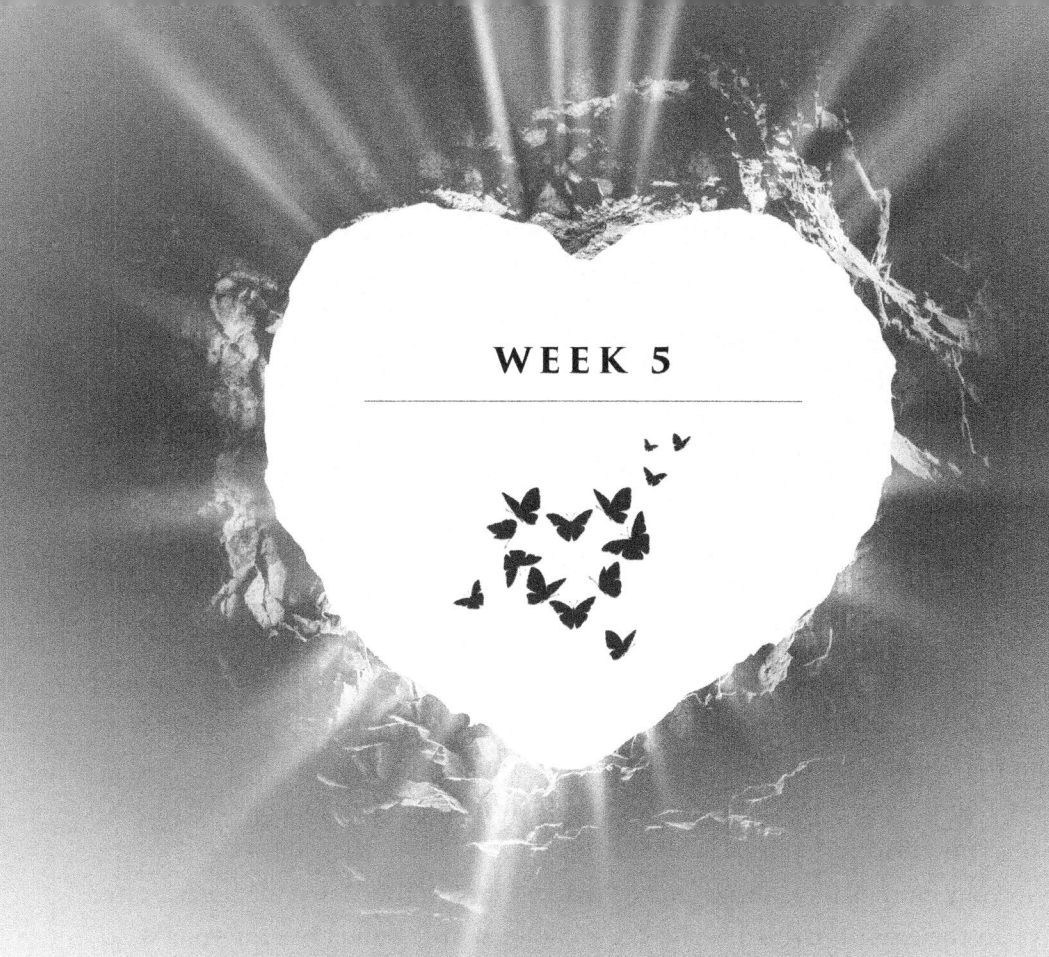

CHAPTER 5: E- Enabling

HERE IS MY PRAYER FOR YOU THIS WEEK:

Father God, we thank You that You are a God of mercy and justice. Forgive us for missing the mark of not following Your Word as we should. Help us to not support an environment of wrong behavior and irresponsibility. Help my sister to not make excuses for her husband or get offended by the truth about herself. You said in Your Word that if we need wisdom to ask You for it, and that You would give it to us. I ask for Your wisdom for my sister right now. Give her what to say as she speaks the truth in love to her husband. Let her know what is just on her behalf. Give her the courage and strength to stand up for righteousness. Help her to love herself and stand for what is right for herself in accordance to how You want her to be cared for. Take away her stony heart and give her a heart that is tender and sensitive to You and others. In Jesus' name I pray. Amen.

This week you will discover the best lens (or scriptures) to look through in the Word of God so that you that you will be able to identify the behaviors of the abuser that you will not help to enable.

In prayer I will lead you to ask God to give you His eternal view, so that He will give you His eternal view of your marriage. I will lead you to ask Him to give you His wisdom to be able to set boundaries that are respectful and consequences that are protective for you.

By the time you finish reading this chapter, you may identify some ways that you have been enabling your husband's abusive behaviors. After I make the blind spot of enabling visible to you, it will no longer be a hindrance, keeping you from standing up for yourself so that you will be respected.

I will challenge you to do several things this week to let your light shine and to put your heart vision into motion.

In your journal, look ahead at the **Perfect Lens** of **The Word** for the next five days. In the space provided, write the Bible verse that you chose for your scripture memory for this week:

_____

_____

_____

_____

_____

Each day read your memory verse for the week first. Then read the scripture for that day before you pray.

DAY 21

GOD'S VIEWPOINT
The Big Picture

In the space below, write your own personal prayer to Father God that you will have wisdom in requiring your husband to take care of his responsibilities so that you will not continue to do them for him. Also ask God to give you wisdom that you will take care of your own responsibilities so that you will be empowered as well.

Father God,

_____

_____

_____

_____

_____

_____

In Jesus' name,

Amen

THE PERFECT LENS – THE WORD

Read Galatians 6:5 (GW)

Assume your own responsibility.

HEART VISION

Close your eyes and look in your heart so that you can see what things you are doing that you would expect your husband to be doing if you were both working on the relationship equally as hard. How does this make you feel? When you open your eyes, write in the space provided what you saw.

_____
_____
_____
_____
_____
_____

You married because of love, but now do you feel that your husband's behavior has hurt you?

_____

In what way?

_____
_____
_____
_____

Day 21

SHINE YOUR LIGHT

Sometimes the relationship is so destroyed by the abuser that there is no repairing it. Is this how your relationship is?

_____

If so, what will you do to make plans to move forward? What legal, residential, and financial issues need to be addressed?

_____
_____
_____

If the abuser is willing to get help and put in the work to be responsible and respect you and your wishes, what will you decide to ask for from your husband that will cause one or more major changes at home?

_____
_____

When is the best time for you to ask him? How will you ask him?

_____
_____

After you ask him, write down whether or not he is willing to do what you asked him to do for the sake of your marriage. Write down what his response was?

_____
_____
_____

Find a behavioral heath therapist in your area who is trained in working with abusive relationships. Write their name here.

_____

Make an appointment for yourself or both of you. Write it here.

_____

_____

No matter what the outcome is, remember that God promises never to leave or forsake you. Remember that He is in control. Also remember that He will work everything out for your good.

DAY 22

GOD'S VIEWPOINT
The Big Picture

In the space below, write your own personal prayer to Father God that you will see how He sees your husband if he is not providing for and taking care of his family in every way – financially, emotionally, spiritually and with his words and deeds.

Father God,

_____
_____
_____
_____
_____
_____
_____
_____

In Jesus' name,

Amen

THE PERFECT LENS – THE WORD

Read 1 Timothy 5:8 (NET)

But if someone does not provide for his own, especially his own family, he has denied the (Christian) faith, and is worse than an unbeliever.

HEART VISION

Close your eyes and look in your heart so that you can see in what ways that your husband is providing for you and what ways your husband is not providing for you in all areas of your life. When you open your eyes, in the space provided write what you saw.

_____
_____
_____
_____
_____

Are you making any excuses for why your husband is acting immature or not being responsible?

_____

If so, what are the excuses?

_____
_____
_____
_____

Are you constantly making your husband a priority, rather than yourself?

___

In what ways?

___
___
___
___

SHINE YOUR LIGHT

What can you do to make yourself a priority this week, and when will you do this?

___
___
___
___
___
___
___
___
___

DAY 23

GOD'S VIEWPOINT
The Big Picture

In the space below, write your own personal prayer to Father God that He will remove the hard heart that has formed over time and replace it with a tender sensitive heart.

Father God,

_____

_____

_____

_____

_____

_____

_____

_____

In Jesus' name,

Amen

THE PERFECT LENS – THE WORD

Read Ezekiel 36:26 NLT

And I will give you a new heart, and I will put a new spirit in you. I will take out your stony, stubborn heart and give you a tender, responsive heart.

HEART VISION

Close your eyes and look in your heart. What does it look and feel like? Does it look hard or soft? Does it feel cold or warm? Is it in pain, or is it healed? Why? When you open your eyes, write in the space provided what you saw.

_____
_____
_____
_____
_____
_____
_____

If I asked you whether YOU are (or ever were) an abused or battered woman, would you immediately feel angry or offended?

_____

Why?

_____
_____
_____

SHINE YOUR LIGHT

Be grateful for His promise. Ask God today for His promise that He will give you a heart that is alive and tender again that is sensitive and can believe once more. He promises to give it to you. You don't have to try to conjure it up. This may be a process that happens a little at a time but expect it. Confess it. Thank Him for it. And continue to give Him praise. Personalize this promise to yourself from God. Finish this sentence: "Thank you God for promising me that You will give me...

_____

_____

_____

_____

_____

_____

_____

DAY 24

GOD'S VIEWPOINT
The Big Picture

In the space below, write your own personal prayer to Father God that He show you whether or not your husband is willing to do what is good for you and his family.

Father God,

_____

_____

_____

_____

_____

_____

_____

In Jesus' name,

Amen

THE PERFECT LENS – THE WORD

Read 2 Thessalonians 3:11-14 (NIV)

The one who is unwilling to work shall not eat. We hear that some among you are idle and disruptive. They are not busy... Such people we command and urge in the Lord Jesus Christ to settle down and earn the food they eat...never tire in doing what is good. Take special note of anyone who does not obey our instruction in this letter. Do not associate with them, in order that they may feel ashamed.

HEART VISION

Close your eyes and look in your heart so that you can see what boundaries that your husband is crossing that is being disrespectful to you. What boundaries need to be put in place so that you will feel safe and secure with expressing your feelings, and him expressing his? Concerning your finances? Concerning your quality time? Concerning household chores? Concerning other friends and family? Concerning your children? Concerning what other issues? When you open your eyes, in the space provided write what you saw.

_____
_____
_____
_____
_____
_____
_____
_____
_____
_____
_____

SHINE YOUR LIGHT

What are you going to do differently if your husband doesn't do what you asked?

_____
_____
_____

Before you talk to your husband, when can you set an appointment to talk to one or both of you support persons that you identified in chapters 1 and 3? Write the appointment time here.

_____
_____
_____

Make an appointment with a professional counselor if you feel that you may be in danger whenever you do decide to talk to your husband about your boundaries and consequences. Write the appointment time here.

_____

Talk with your support team about the boundaries and consequences that you want for yourself and ask your support person(s) to help you make a safe plan to ask for a change that you want.

Let them know that you need a plan in case you have to face negative consequences if your husband doesn't agree to your suggested change. Let one or both of your support people know when you are planning on talking to your husband.

DAY 25

GOD'S VIEWPOINT
The Big Picture

In the space below, write your own personal prayer to Father God that He will reveal to you those things that are not pure and not good and not full of truth and light in your relationship. Ask God to give you wisdom to know what to do, so that you will not have to continue to deal with them in the future.

Father God,

_____
_____
_____
_____
_____
_____
_____

In Jesus' name,

Amen

Day 25

THE PERFECT LENS – THE WORD

Read Ephesians 5:11 (NIV)

Have nothing to do with the fruitless deeds of darkness, but rather expose them.

HEART VISION

Close your eyes and look in your heart so that you can see what you need to do if your husband refuses to respect what you want him to do to save your marriage. When you open your eyes, in the space provided write down what you saw.

_____
_____
_____
_____
_____
_____
_____
_____

Are you ready to face the consequences of your husband's not wanting to adhere to your boundaries?

_____
_____

Do you feel that you and your children are worth more than what you may have to sacrifice in order to have the life that you deserve?

_____
_____

SHINE YOUR LIGHT

When can you set a good time and in what safe public place (that you can drive to and from separately from your husband if necessary) can you go to discuss your boundaries with your husband and let him know what you will do if he does not agree to them?

_____
_____
_____

Let your husband know about your support person. If he dismisses what you have to say, let him know that you are sorry he feels that way, and leave. Ask your support person to either be there at your meeting place at a distance, to call to check on you every ten minutes, or allow you and your children to spend the night if necessary.

Write down the outcome of this meeting.

_____
_____
_____

When can you set up a follow-up meeting with your support person(s) to make sure you are following through with your consequences?

_____
_____
_____

WEEK 5 NOTES

Week 5 Notes

WEEK 6

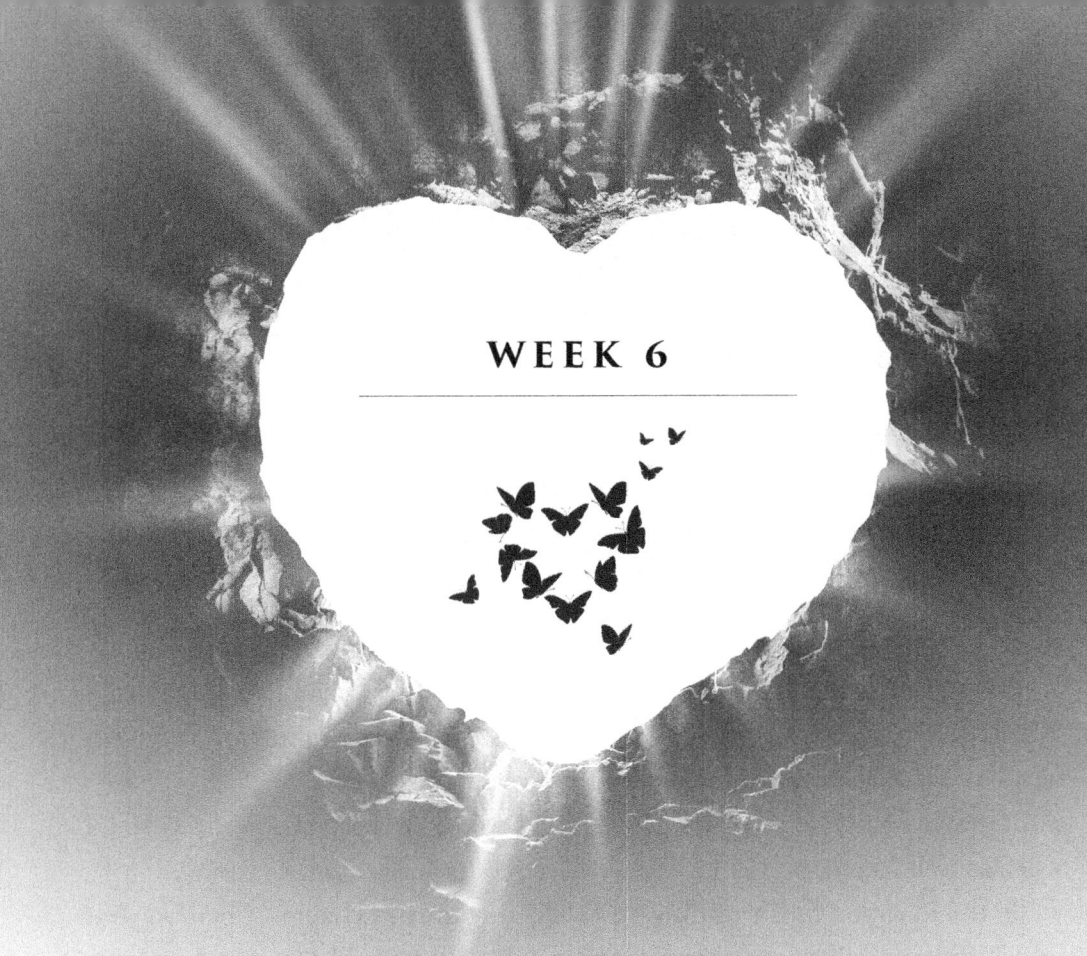

CHAPTER 5: E- Esteem

HERE IS MY PRAYER FOR YOU THIS WEEK:

Father God, You are Elohim, the God that creates. Thank You for creating our spirits and creating us in your image. Thank You that in Your kingdom our rank is right under the angels.

Thank You for adopting us in Your kingdom when we believe in Your Son, Jesus. Thank You for making us a part of Your royal priesthood. I pray for my sister that she agrees with Your Word that You made her wonderful and beautiful.

As a believer, I pray she receives the revelation that she is Your daughter and a daughter of Zion. I pray that as she understands her spirit of nobility and ex-

cellence, she will with confidence walk in her authority as a daughter of Sarah. And then help her not to throw away her confidence.

Thank You for giving her the spirit of love, power, and a strong mind. Help her to be Godly-proud of herself, and to believe in herself. Be the lifter of her head.

Help her to love, stand up for, and look out for herself. Help her to be strong and courageous. Give her the courage to make the right decisions that will bring needed change in her life and in the lives of her children. Lead her to the right people who will be an advocate for her. Protect her from all hurt, harm, and danger. All these things I ask in your Son Jesus' name. Amen

This week you will discover the best lens (or scriptures) to look through in the Word of God so that low esteem will not cause you to have a distorted view of who you actually are and what God wants you to do.

In prayer I will lead you to ask God to give you His eternal view of yourself. I will also lead you to ask Him to help you see yourself like He sees you.

By the time you finish reading and reflecting on this chapter, I believe your self-confidence will have grown more than it is right now. I hope that *not believing* in yourself will *no longer* be the blind spot that will hold you back from what God wants you to do. He wants you to be true to yourself. He wants you to take care of yourself and your children so that your lives will truly glorify Him.

I will challenge you to do several things this week to let your light shine and to put your heart vision into motion.

In your journal look ahead at the **Perfect Lens** of **The Word** for the next five days. In the space provided, write the Bible verse that you chose for your scripture memory for this week:

_____

_____

_____

_____

Each day read your memory verse for the week first. Then read the scripture for that day before you pray.

DAY 26

GOD'S VIEWPOINT
The Big Picture

In the space below, write your own personal prayer to Father God who is the King over all kings. Thank Him for adopting you into His royal family and making you His precious daughter, His princess, and the apple of His eye. As a queen has dominion and has authority to rule and reign, so He has given you this authority to do so in your world around you. Thank Him for that right now.

Father God,

_____

_____

_____

_____

_____

_____

_____

In Jesus' name,

Amen

THE PERFECT LENS – THE WORD

Read Revelations 5:10 NKJV

And You have made us (God's children) kings (and queens), and priests to our God; And we shall reign on the earth.

HEART VISION

Close your eyes and look in your heart so that you can see the beauty and order that exists in heaven. God promises that He is preparing mansions for us. When you look with your heart, how do you see your mansion? Now look with your heart and see your home. What does it look like compared to what your future home in heaven will look like? I'm not referring to expensive things – only the creativity of what you have–creating an atmosphere that is clean and in order, like we mentioned on Day 6. When you open your eyes, in the space provided write what you saw.

_____
_____
_____
_____
_____
_____
_____
_____
_____

Because you are a daughter of Sarah with a spirit of excellence, beauty and order, what changes would you like to make in your living quarters to reflect your royal heavenly qualities? How can you bring beauty and order to your home so that it looks like heaven on earth? What can you do to make your angels feel comfortable–like they are in their heavenly home–as they hover around your home?

_____
_____
_____
_____
_____
_____

SHINE YOUR LIGHT

What are you going **to clean first** to make your living quarters fit for a queen?

_____
_____
_____
_____

What are you going **to put in order first** to make your living quarters fit for a queen?

_____
_____
_____
_____

DAY 27

GOD'S VIEWPOINT
The Big Picture

In the space below, write your own personal prayer to Father God thanking Him for making you so awesome and wonderful.

Father God,

_____
_____
_____
_____
_____
_____
_____
_____

In Jesus' name,

Amen

THE PERFECT LENS – THE WORD

Read Psalms 139:14 NHEB

I will give thanks to you, for I am awesomely and wonderfully made. Your works are wonderful. My soul knows that very well.

HEART VISION

Close your eyes and look in your heart so that you can see all the ways that make you awesome and to see what makes you so wonderful. Don't allow negative thoughts to linger in this exercise. Concentrate only on positive thoughts about yourself. What do you love about yourself? When you open your eyes, in the space provided write what you saw.

SHINE YOUR LIGHT

It is easy to listen to the negative thoughts about yourself that come to your mind. These bad thoughts will definitely come, but you can decide whether or not to dwell on them. I encourage you to stop beating up on yourself! Start today being intentional about dwelling only on good thoughts about yourself.

When you do this exercise remember this scripture: "Finally, brothers (and sisters), whatever things are true, whatever things are honorable, whatever things are just, whatever things are pure, whatever things are lovely, whatever things are of good report; if there is any praise, think about these things." Philippians 4:8.

For this exercise write down as many positive affirmation statements about yourself as you can, then say them out loud so that you can hear them. Write positive statements about yourself, even if you don't feel like it is true right now. Write them as an act of faith that God will help you to see them become a reality in the near future. Say these to yourself every morning when you wake up. (Let me give you some examples: I am beautiful. I am strong. I am capable. I am smart.) Now it's your turn.

_____

_____

_____

_____

_____

_____

_____

_____

_____

_____

DAY 28

GOD'S VIEWPOINT
The Big Picture

In the space below, write your own personal prayer to Father God to help you to love yourself. Ask God to help you to love yourself so much that you will not allow anyone to continue to mistreat you again. Also ask God to help you to forgive yourself for anything that you have been feeling guilty about that you feel that you should not have done.

Father God,

_____

_____

_____

_____

_____

_____

_____

In Jesus' name,

Amen

THE PERFECT LENS – THE WORD

Read Matthew 37-39 GNT

*Jesus answered him, "Love the Lord your God with all your heart, with all your soul, and with all your mind. This is the greatest and most important commandment." The Second Commandment is similar to it: "Love your neighbor as you **love yourself**."*

HEART VISION

Close your eyes and look in your heart so that you can see those things that you love. What are the things that you like and would want for yourself? Think of yourself as a dear friend. What would you do to treat – you? How would you celebrate yourself? In the space provided, when you open your eyes, write what you saw.

_____
_____
_____
_____
_____
_____

What scented candles, oils, perfumes, and lotions do you like and would want?

_____
_____
_____
_____

SHINE YOUR LIGHT

Because you love yourself, what will you stop allowing your partner to continue to do to you that is disrespectful?

___

How and when are you going to communicate this boundary to him?*

___

What consequence will you give if this boundary is crossed?*

___

* *Utilize your support team the same way as you did on Day 25 if needed.*

Because you love yourself, give yourself a "just because" treat this week. What will it be?

_____

_____

_____

_____

When will you celebrate yourself?

_____

DAY 29

GOD'S VIEWPOINT
The Big Picture

Woman of God, you are beautiful. Remember we discussed this on Day 14. Don't let your negative thoughts and feelings about yourself dismiss this truth. In the space below, write your own personal prayer to Father God to remind you of how beautiful your heart and spirit is, and ask Him to give you the desire to show how beautiful you are on the outside. In prayer, ask God to help you reflect your inward beauty as He helps you to make a special effort to look cute when you face the world each day.

Father God,

_____

_____

_____

_____

_____

In Jesus' name,

Amen

The Perfect Lens – The Word

Read about Queen Esther: Esther 2:12b NIV

She had to complete twelve months of beauty treatments prescribed for the women, six months with oil of myrrh and six with perfumes and cosmetics.

Heart Vision

Close your eyes and in your heart see how you would look if you were given a makeover that was fit for a queen. How would your hair, makeup, clothes, shoes, and accessories look? When you open your eyes, in the space below describe how you saw yourself.

_____

_____

_____

_____

Have you been giving yourself special attention to make sure your hair and makeup is done?

_____

Why or why not?

_____

_____

_____

_____

Have you went shopping for yourself to get a cute outfit, shoes, or accessories lately?

_____

Why or why not?

_____
_____
_____
_____
_____
_____

Have you had a spa day lately?

_____

Why or why not?

_____
_____
_____
_____
_____

If cost is a factor, consider getting soothing oils and sweet, smelling lotion from other places. (i.e. Bath and Body Works or even The Dollar Tree).

SHINE YOUR LIGHT

What will you start doing to make a special effort to look cute each day?

_____
_____
_____

What appointment will you make for yourself to have a makeover in one area?

_____

Write down with whom and when you made this appointment.

_____
_____

When are you going shopping next for yourself?

_____

For what are you going shopping for?

_____

DAY 30

GOD'S VIEWPOINT
The Big Picture

In the space below, write your own prayer to Father God help you to make your desires a priority. Ask God to either remind you of or give you your own personal, tangible dream for yourself. Ask God to give you a vision for a reachable goal that you can set for yourself in a realistic time frame.

Father God,

___

___

___

___

___

___

___

___

In Jesus' name,

Amen

THE PERFECT LENS – THE WORD

Read Proverbs 29:18a KJV

Where there is no vision, the people perish.

HEART VISION

Close your eyes and look in your heart so that you can see one thing in which you know is obtainable that you want for yourself that you can physically touch. *(This is different from the dream that you saw in your heart on Day 19 of a bright future that you want for your life and relationships. These are intangible.)* When you open your eyes, in the space provided write what you saw.

_____

_____

_____

_____

_____

Is this a one-year, five-year, or ten-year goal?

_____

Explain what has kept you from pursuing this goal?

_____

_____

_____

_____

_____

_____

SHINE YOUR LIGHT

What can you do to make a step toward bringing to reality the tangible dream that you wrote down in your heart vision exercise?

_____
_____
_____
_____
_____

When will you do this?

_____

WEEK 6 NOTES

Week 6 Notes

WEEK 7

CHAPTER 7:
Moving Forward to Your Purpose

Forgiveness is a key part of you being able to move forward to your purpose. Here is a simple prayer that you can pray in your **Shine Your Light** exercise* on Day 31, if you need to forgive your abuser:

Father God, thank You for being the God who sees. Thank You for being so good to me. Thank You for caring so much about me and how my heart has been hurt. You know the pain that I have felt because of (tell God the reasons for all of the pain and hurt that you have). Right now, I release and cast all of this hurt and pain at your feet, God.

Thank You, Jesus for dying on the cross for my sins, and I make a choice to forgive (his name) as an act of my free will. I reject all thoughts of revenge for (his name). I release my right to hold him accountable to me. I trust You, God that in Your own time and way, You will take care of (his name) according to Your will. Thank You, Holy Spirit for giving me Your power to forgive so that I can have freedom. All of these things I ask in Jesus' name. Amen.

Here is my prayer for you this week:

Father God, I thank You that You are Love. You are faithful, just, and full of mercy. As my sister seeks You on the direction she is to take in her life, I thank You that You order her steps. Thank You for being the Lord who is her shepherd. Because You are her Shepherd, You lead and guide her. I thank You that she shall not want any good thing, because You will give her what she desires, and help her to be content.

Thank You for supplying the finances and material needs that she needs for herself and her children while she goes through this time in her life. Connect her with the right people at the right time that will be there to support her and her children. Protect her and her children.

Thank You for revealing to her which way You want her to go in her spirit. At any time that she may fall, I thank You that You are always right there to pick her up. Help her to forgive herself and others who may offend her. I thank You for the plans that You have for her bright future.

Whatever her life purpose or destiny is, reveal it to her spirit. Confirm it with two or three witnesses. I thank You that every good work that You begin in her You will complete it. I thank You for opening the eyes of her spirit so that by faith she will see herself and others like You do. All these things I ask in Jesus' name. Amen.

This week you will discover the best lens (or scriptures) to look through in the Word of God so that you will move forward with your life purpose.

I will lead you to pray to that God will help you to forgive not only your abuser, but yourself and give you His eternal view of your path to a brighter future.

By the time you finish reading this chapter you will understand the importance of forgiveness and how it frees you up to fulfill your destiny.

I will challenge you to do several things this week to let your light shine and to put your heart vision into motion.

In your journal look ahead at the **Perfect Lens** of **The Word** for the next five days. In the space provided, write the Bible verse that you chose for your scripture memory for this week:

_____
_____
_____
_____
_____

Each day read your memory verse for the week first. Then read the scripture for that day before you pray.

DAY 31

GOD'S VIEWPOINT
The Big Picture

In the space below, write your own prayer to Father God that He will help you to identity any unforgiveness that you may have in your heart for yourself and/or your abuser and to help you to go through the process of forgiveness in order for you to be free from the bondage of unforgiveness.

Father God,

_____
_____
_____
_____
_____
_____
_____
_____

In Jesus' name,

Amen

THE PERFECT LENS – THE WORD

Read Matthew 6:14-15 (NLT)

If you forgive men when they sin against you, your heavenly Father will also forgive you. But if you do not forgive men their sins, your Father will not forgive your sins.

HEART VISION

I know this exercise is not easy, but it needs to be done so that you can move forward. Close your eyes and look with your heart to see who you need to forgive and what they have done that you need to forgive. When you open your eyes, in the space provided write what you saw.

_____
_____
_____
_____
_____

Is there anything that you need to forgive yourself for?

_____

If so, What?

_____
_____
_____
_____
_____

SHINE YOUR LIGHT

Are you going to make a decision to forgive and release your right to hold a grudge for those in your "Heart Vision" exercise, including yourself?

_____

If no, Why?

_____

_____

_____

_____

_____

Ask God to help you with making this decision. Continue to seek God for His help so that you can be free and move forward.

If yes, you can pray your own prayer of forgiveness or the one at the beginning of this week's journal exercise. * If the prayer is for yourself just substitute (his name) for (myself or me) in the prayer.

After you sincerely pray this prayer, thank and praise God for your deliverance and continue to go through the process of refusing to dwell on negative thoughts about yourself or your abuser each day. Pray for grace for yourself and your abuser. Then accept God's new mercy every morning.

DAY 32

GOD'S VIEWPOINT
The Big Picture

In the space below, write your own personal prayer to Father God that He will help you to make the best decision for yourself and your children concerning your marriage or your intimate relationship.

Father God,

_____

_____

_____

_____

_____

_____

_____

In Jesus' name,

Amen

THE PERFECT LENS – THE WORD

Read Proverbs 3:6

Remember the Lord in everything you do, and He will show you the right way.

HEART VISION

Close your eyes and look in your heart so that you can see what God is showing you to do concerning your marriage. What is your heart saying? What do you just know in your gut? The Word of God says out of your belly shall flow rivers of living water. (John 7:38) The Holy Spirit is the living water, and out of your core (where your spirit lives) is where He flows from. Do not listen to all the reasoning thoughts in your head. When you open your eyes, in the space provided write what you saw.

_____
_____
_____
_____

Are you ready to make a decision to change your life?

_____

Why or why not?

_____
_____
_____
_____

SHINE YOUR LIGHT

If you did not see what God is showing you what you should do concerning your marriage, ask God to give you His promise found in your scripture today that He will show you the right way. Continue to thank Him for showing you before you get His revelation as an act of faith.

If you are not ready to make a decision, make an appointment with a professional behavior health therapist trained in abusive relationships. They can help you to get self-help until you are ready to make a decision. Write your appointment time and place here.

_____

Remember also that God gives you the power to use your own free will to make decisions you want for yourself. Sometimes God is waiting on you to step out on faith and believe that He loves you enough and that He will supply all of your needs. If you delight in Him, He promises to give you the desires of your heart. (Psalm 37:4) What do you want?

_____
_____
_____

God may never part the clouds of the heavens and show you a miraculous sign. Know that as His child, God wants the best for you. I encourage you to trust and believe that your Father God will give you wisdom. Trust Him to do the things that you, His daughter, cannot do. Watch Him move. If you were not worried about making a mistake, what would your gut decision be?

_____
_____
_____
_____

DAY 33

GOD'S VIEWPOINT
The Big Picture

In the space below, write your own personal prayer to Father God that He will guide you each step of the way as you take care of yourself and move forward to your brighter future.

Father God,

_____
_____
_____
_____
_____
_____
_____
_____

In Jesus' name,

Amen

THE PERFECT LENS – THE WORD

Read Proverb 16:9 (ISV)

A person plans his (her) way, but the Lord directs his (her) steps.

HEART VISION

Close your eyes and look in your heart so that you can see what your next step should be if you decide to make a transition from your marriage. See what your next step should be if you are not ready for this but want to look out for yourself so that you guard your emotions, mental status, and physical safety and that of your children. When you open your eyes, in the space provided write what you saw.

_____
_____
_____
_____
_____
_____

What is your own plan of transition or self care and safety even without your heart vision?

_____
_____
_____
_____
_____
_____

SHINE YOUR LIGHT

You can exercise your authority as a believer to use your God-given free will to decide to move on from an abusive marriage or relationship. Whether with or without seeing with your heart, God still promises to direct your steps in the scripture for today. I encourage you to step out on faith and start moving. What are you doing to do first to put your plan into action?

_____
_____
_____
_____
_____

If you need help with a plan, contact one of the resources in appendix B, your behavioral health therapist, or your support team. When will you contact them?

_____

When are you going to put your plan into action?

_____
_____
_____
_____
_____

Continue to be sensitive to your spirit as God redirects your plans as you go.

DAY 34

GOD'S VIEWPOINT
The Big Picture

In the space below, write your own personal prayer to Father God that as you work your plan, God will supply everything that you need for you plan to succeed.

Father God,

_____
_____
_____
_____
_____
_____
_____

In Jesus' name,

Amen

THE PERFECT LENS – THE WORD

Read Philippians 4:19 (NIV)

And my God will meet all your needs according to the riches of his glory in Christ Jesus.

HEART VISION

Close your eyes and look in your heart so that you can see yourself having everything that you need for your transition plan to be successful in just a few months from now. When you open your eyes, in the space provided write what you saw.

_____
_____
_____
_____
_____
_____

What are the immediate things that you need to make your transition happen?

_____
_____
_____
_____
_____

SHINE YOUR LIGHT

List the resources that can help you during your transition from appendix B.

_____
_____
_____
_____
_____

Ask for help from your support team. What can they help you with?

_____
_____
_____
_____
_____

Find out what other community organizations can help you with. (i.e. police, women's legal services, primary care providers, social services, shelters, etc). What did you find out?

_____
_____
_____
_____
_____

DAY 35

GOD'S VIEWPOINT
The Big Picture

In the space below, write your own personal prayer to Father God that He will lead you to your true purpose in life when you are free of abuse.

Father God,

___

___

___

___

___

___

___

___

___

In Jesus' name,

Amen

THE PERFECT LENS – THE WORD

Read Exodus 9:16 (NIV)

But I have raised you up for this very purpose, that I might show you My power and that My name might be proclaimed in all the earth.

HEART VISION

Close your eyes and look in your heart so that you can see yourself fulfilling your destiny by helping others. When you open your eyes, in the space provided write what you saw.

_____
_____
_____
_____
_____

Do you know exactly what your life purpose is?

_____

If so, What?

_____
_____
_____
_____
_____

SHINE YOUR LIGHT

If you don't know your life purpose, will you commit to reading **A Purpose-Driven Life** by Rick Warren?

_____

If you do know your life purpose that will in some way help others, what step or steps can you take to make it happen?

_____
_____
_____
_____
_____
_____
_____
_____
_____
_____
_____
_____

Congratulations! You did it! You finished your **Heart Vision** journaling, but start your next devotional book that you were to purchase/order on Day 16. I encourage you to continue looking with your heart.

WEEK 7 NOTES

Week 7 Notes

gfv
...because sight matters.

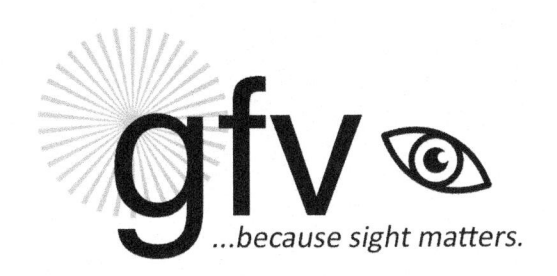

GIVE 1

One dollar is donated to charity for every copy of *Heart Vision Journal* that is sold. This charitable organization is **Great Faith Vision**.

Great Faith Vision needs your help!

They need *your help* to further their mission to provide both **physical and spiritual vision** by spreading the Good News of the Gospel and providing eye care services, eyeglasses, and medical care (including surgery and medications) to those without access or without the means to afford these services in the USA and around the world.

Great Faith Vision partners with host pastors, missionaries, and community organizations, including shelters, to open doors to the Gospel by providing these services to their communities.

Great Faith Vision is dependent on volunteers, prayers, and financial support of people like you who share their passion.

To give on-line go to:
www.gfv.org

GFV is an all-volunteer, faith based, 501 (c) 3 tax exempt non-profit. All donations to this charity are tax deductible.

Thank you

About the Author

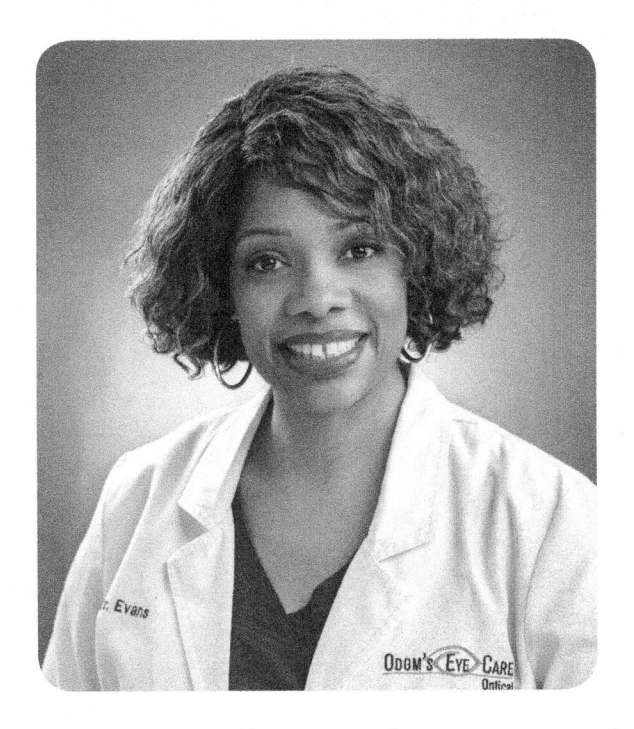

DR. DELLIA EVANS is a well-respected optometrist who has helped over 250,000 patients to improve their vision for over 25 years. Dr. Dellia helps people to see more clearly both physically and spiritually. She earned a B.A. Cum Laude from the University of Mississippi and a Doctor of Optometry degree from The University of Alabama at Birmingham. A resident of Jackson, Mississippi, she is happily re-married and has two adult children and one granddaughter.

Made in the USA
Columbia, SC
20 September 2020